FERTILITY COOKBOOK FOR COUPLES

Curated fun, delicious, and healthy Recipes for improving fertility and preparing for pregnancy

LISA BRITT

FERTILITY COOKBOOK FOR COUPLES............ 0
Chapter 1: Understanding Fertility...................... 9
Chapter 2:The science behind the fertility diet 16
    FOODS TO EAT FOR HIM AND FOR HER.... 19
Chapter 3: Breakfasts..28
Chapter Four: Lunch.. 44
    Fertility protein Bowl...............................44
Chapter 5: DINNER... 61
Chapter 6: Desserts and Drinks....................... 73
    Desserts..73
    DRINKS..88
CONCLUSION 95

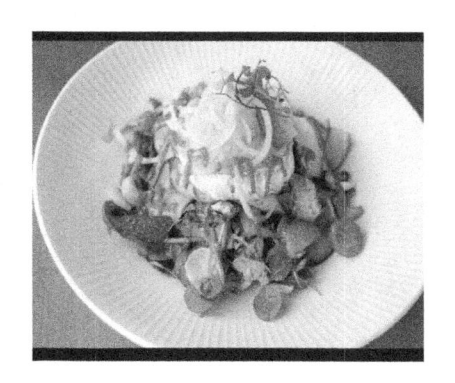

Copyright © [2023] [LISA BRITT].

All rights reserved. No part of this publication may be reproduced, stored in a retrieval system, or transmitted in any form or by any means, electronic, mechanical, photocopying, recording, or otherwise, without the prior written permission of the author.

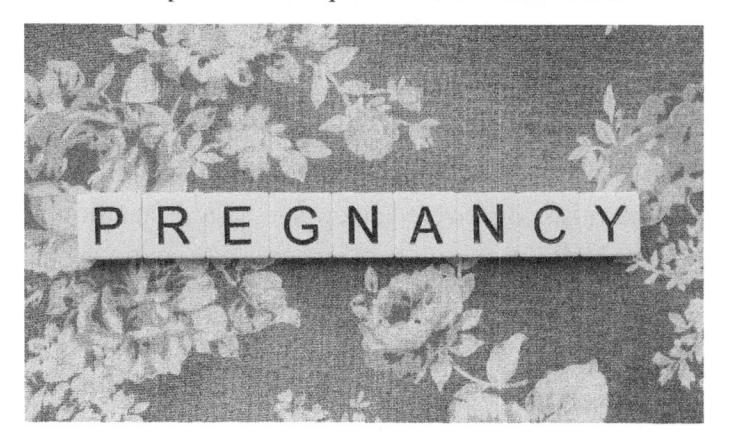

INTRODUCTION

For almost two years, Lisa and her husband had struggled with infertility. They had attempted several different treatments during that period, including a couple cycles of in-vitro fertilization. They had tried their hardest to conceive a child, but had been unsuccessful.

Lisa once discovered a cookbook for couples on fertility. The thought that her diet might affect her ability to conceive piqued her interest. She made the decision to give it a shot and started to make the foods listed in the cookbook.

Lisa was initially skeptical. Yet as she started to follow the food recommendations, she saw that her energy levels and general wellbeing had changed. She also discovered that she could handle the responsibilities of her career and continue her reproductive treatments as planned.

Lisa was shocked at the improvements she obtained from merely modifying her diet. She was so motivated by her achievement that she made the decision to create her own cookbook for couples on fertility.

The recipes Lisa found to be most helpful while she and her husband were trying to conceive are shared in this cookbook along with her personal experience. She also offers advice on how to stay optimistic throughout the procedure and get the most out of fertility treatments.

For couples trying to conceive, Lisa thinks a good diet is crucial. And that's why she created her cookbook: to assist other infertility-affected couples in finding a means to improve their nutrition and way of life.

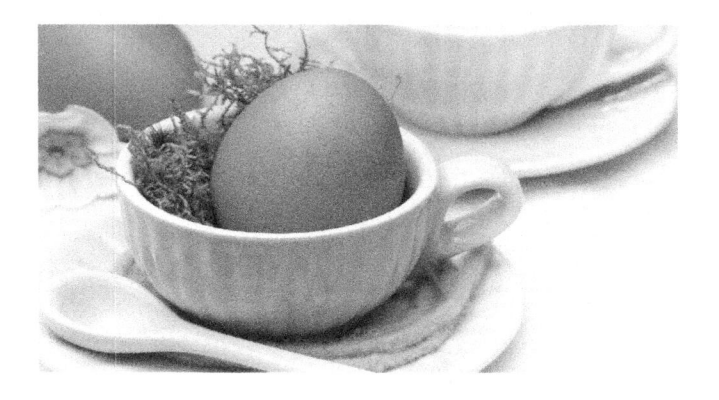

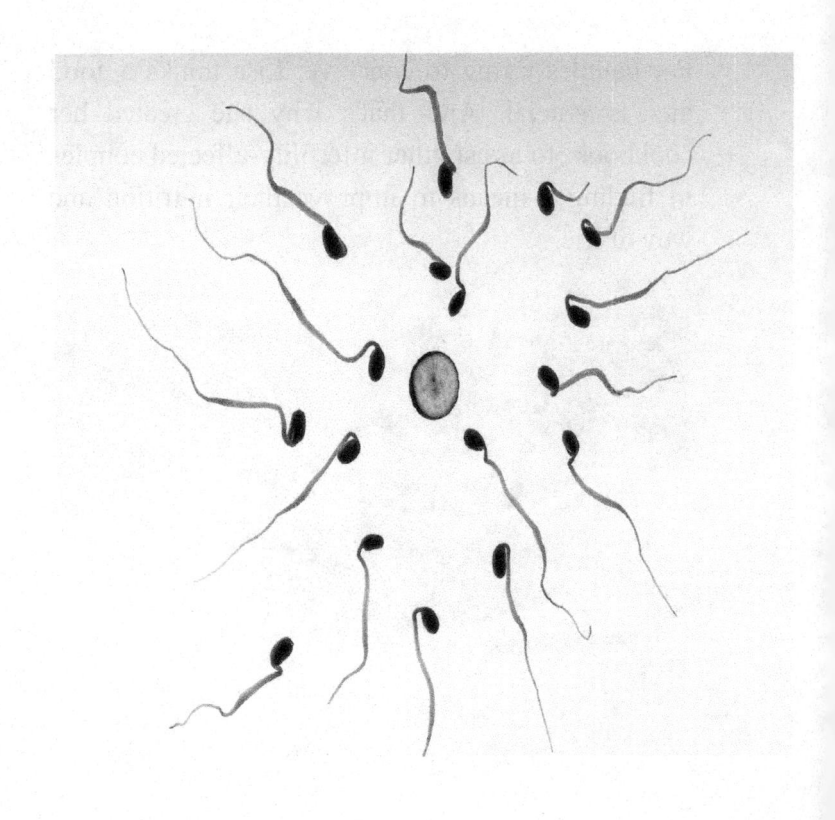

Chapter 1: Understanding Fertility

The capacity to get pregnant and have a child is known as fertility. It is a natural process that can be accelerated by gaining a basic grasp of fertility and altering one's lifestyle.

Timing is the most crucial element in fertility. The days of the month that a woman is most fertile, which are often the days preceding and including ovulation, are when she is most likely to become pregnant. Ovulation, which happens about 14 days before the beginning of a woman's menstrual cycle, is the release of an egg from the ovary. The average menstrual cycle for women is 28 days long, though it might differ from woman to woman. In order to determine when you are most likely to become pregnant, it is vital to chart your cycle and understand the indications of ovulation.

Lifestyle elements can affect fertility in addition to time. Fertility can be enhanced by following a good diet, abstaining from smoking and excessive alcohol use, maintaining a healthy weight, and lowering stress. Exercise is also useful, since it can assist balance hormones and enhance blood flow to the reproductive organs.

By knowing the principles of fertility and implementing lifestyle changes, couples can boost their chances of becoming pregnant and having a safe pregnancy. A fertility cookbook can be a useful tool since it offers scrumptious meals and advice to assist couples in maximizing their fertility.

Finally, it's crucial to comprehend the fundamentals of fertility therapies. Couples may need to think about fertility treatments like in vitro fertilization (IVF), intrauterine insemination (IUI), or donor eggs/sperm depending on the cause of infertility. Before choosing a course of action, it is crucial to talk with a doctor about the dangers and benefits of these treatments because they can be pricey and involved.

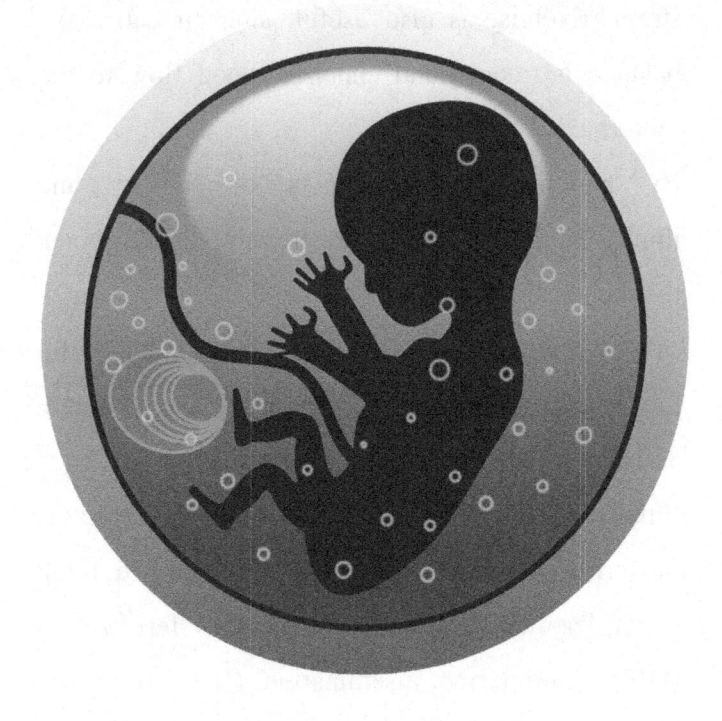

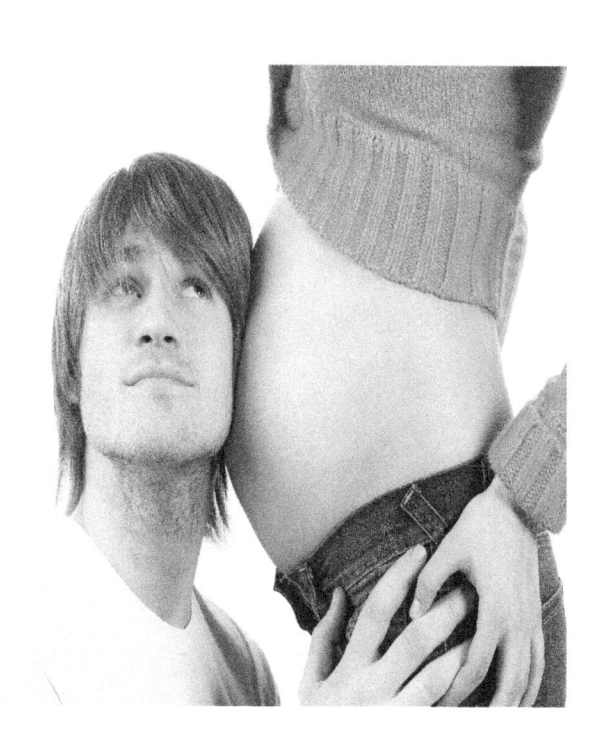

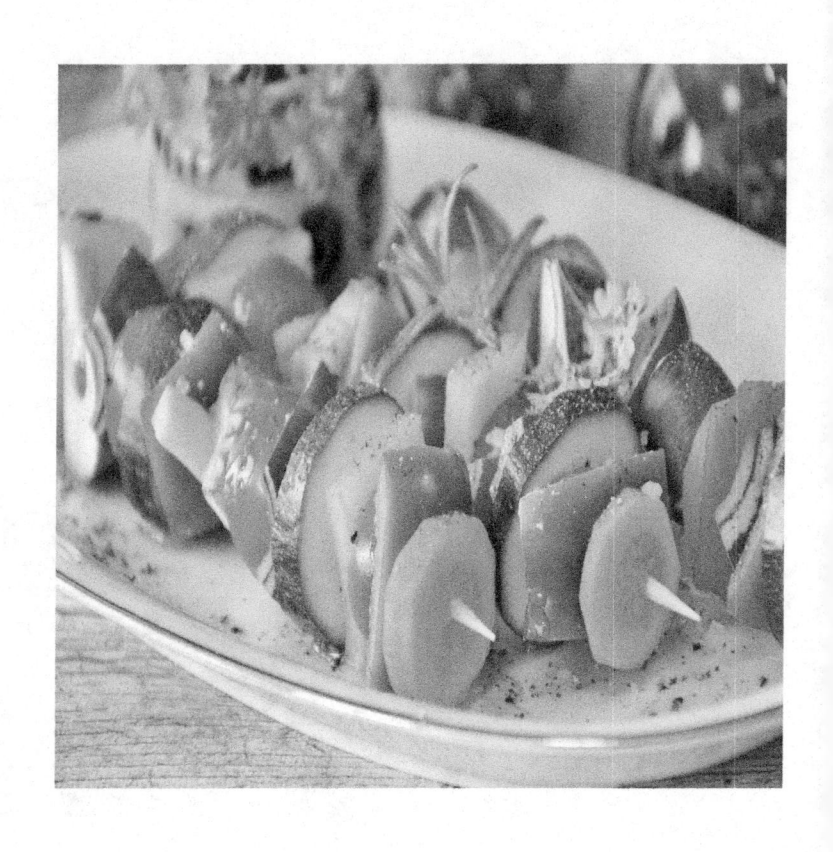

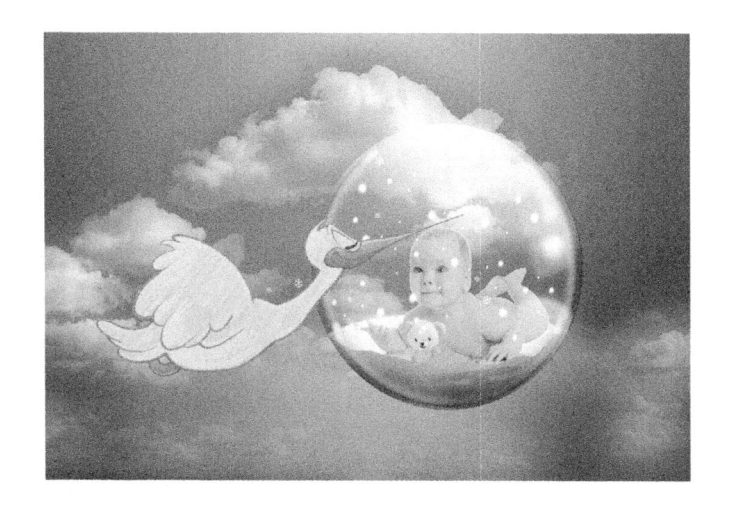

Chapter 2: The science behind the fertility diet

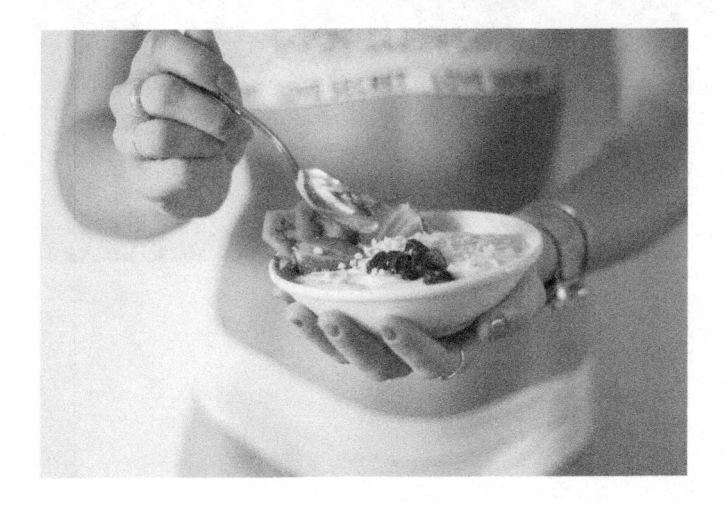

The Fertility Diet is a nutritional strategy to raise conception rates by enhancing both men's and women's reproductive health. It is based on empirical evidence showing that specific dietary and lifestyle choices might enhance fertility. The diet is predicated on the idea that while some foods may be harmful to reproductive health, others may be healthy. The eating of unprocessed, entire foods such fruits, vegetables, whole grains, healthy fats, and lean proteins is emphasized. Also, it advises decreasing trans fats, trans sugars, alcohol, and caffeine consumption.

The diet also promotes alterations to one's way of living, such as lessening stress, steppin up physical exercise, and getting enough sleep. It is believed that these changes will optimize hormone levels and enhance reproductive health.

The considerable clinical research on the fertility diet has shown that it increases fertility in both men and women. According to studies, food can enhance ovarian function, lower the chance of miscarriage, and lower the likelihood of birth abnormalities. It has also been linked to a decreased risk of endometriosis and polycystic ovarian syndrome (PCOS).

Overall, it has been demonstrated that the Fertility Diet improves reproductive health and increases the likelihood of pregnancy. It is predicated on the notion that some food and lifestyle changes may have a favorable effect on fertility. It places a strong emphasis on eating whole, unprocessed foods and steering clear of refined foods, processed foods, alcohol, caffeine, and trans fats. It also promotes lifestyle changes including lessening stress, steppin up physical activity, and obtaining enough sleep.

FOODS TO EAT FOR HIM AND FOR HER

For Him:

1. **Leafy Greens**: The vital vitamins and minerals found in leafy greens can help increase male fertility. The folate found in leafy greens like spinach, kale, and Swiss chard is crucial for the health of sperm.

2. **Nuts**: Nuts are an excellent source of protein and healthy fats, both of which are crucial for the wellbeing of sperm. Essential vitamins and minerals including vitamin E, zinc, and selenium, which are good for fertility, are found in almonds, walnuts, and sunflower seeds.

3. **Whole Grains**: Whole grains are a good source of B vitamins, which might increase male fertility. Oatmeal and barley are excellent providers of folate, which is crucial for the health of sperm.

4. **Eggs**: Packed with choline, B6, B12, and D vitamins as well as protein, eggs are a fertility powerhouse. The B vitamins are crucial for male reproductive health, and choline aids in the creation of healthy sperm.

5. **Spinach**: A B vitamin called folate, which is abundant in spinach, can increase male fertility. Moreover, it has magnesium and zinc, both of which may increase sperm count.

6. **Oysters**: Oysters are rich in zinc, which is necessary for producing healthy sperm. Moreover, zinc supports the production of testosterone, which raises libido.

7. **Fish**: Omega-3 fatty acids can be found in fish including salmon, mackerel, and tuna. These

beneficial lipids might enhance the quality and mobility of sperm.

8.**Avocados**: Avocados are high in beneficial lipids that may enhance the quality and motility of sperm. They also include vitamin E, which aids in sperm damage prevention.

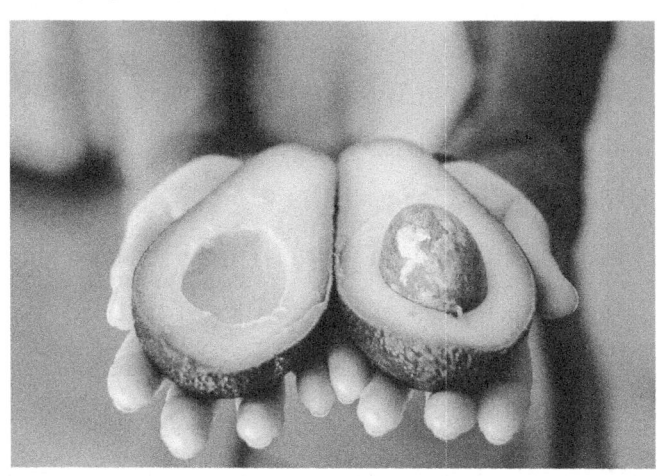

Things She Should Eat:

1. **Berries**: Berries are rich in antioxidants, which can aid in preventing damage to the eggs and reproductive organs.
2. **Leafy Greens**: Kale, spinach, and Swiss chard are a few examples of leafy greens that are high in folate. In addition to lowering the chance of birth abnormalities, folate aids in the production of healthy eggs.
3. **Fish**: Fish strong in omega-3 fatty acids include tuna, mackerel, and salmon. These beneficial fats can help with hormone balance, inflammation control, and egg quality.
4. **Beans**: Beans are a wonderful source of folate and other nutrients. Examples include lentils, kidney beans, and black beans. They can aid in enhancing egg quality and lowering the chance of birth abnormalities.

5.**Nuts**: Nuts, such almonds and walnuts, are rich in protein, vitamins, and minerals as well as heart-healthy fats. These foods can increase fertility and help with hormone balance.

6. **Olive Oil**: Olive oil is full of good lipids that can balance hormones and boost fertility. Antioxidants included in it can shield the reproductive organs from harm.

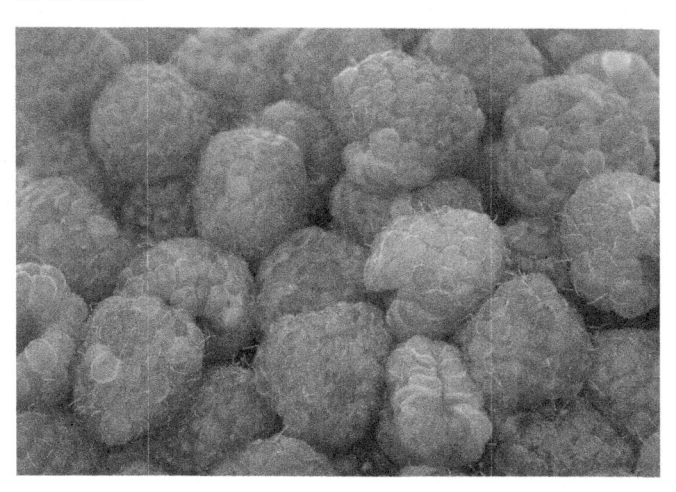

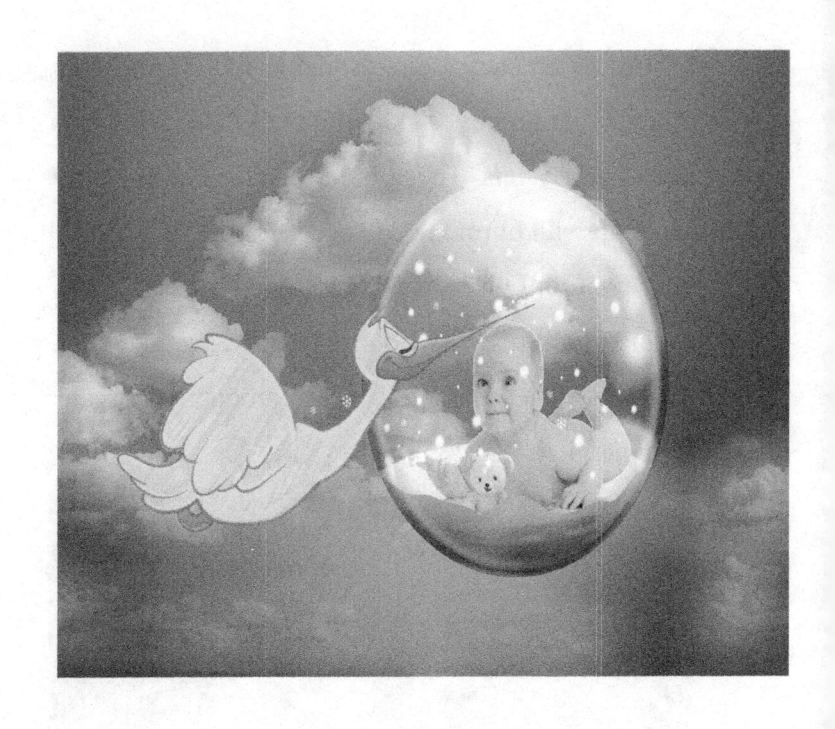

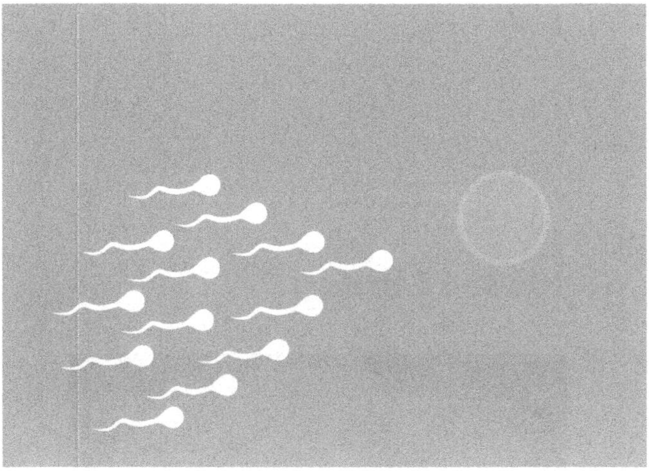

Chapter 3: Breakfasts

Avocado and Egg toast

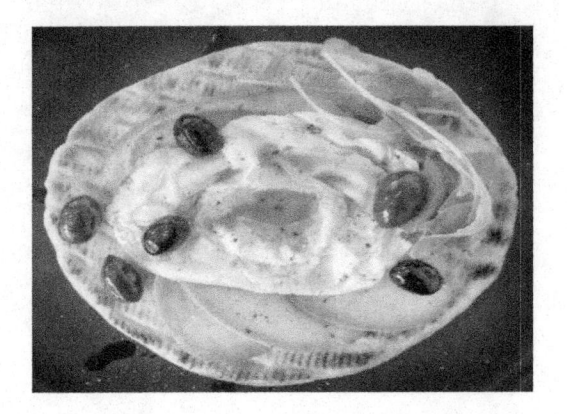

A healthy and scrumptious breakfast like avocado and egg toast is a wonderful way to start the day. A balanced intake of fiber, vitamins, minerals, healthy fats, and proteins from this mixture of foods helps maintain a healthy reproductive system. This dish is simple to prepare and offers a well-rounded meal that can assist to nourish the body for a busy day, making it a fantastic alternative for couples trying to conceive as a breakfast option.

Start by toasting two slices of whole grain bread for the avocado and egg toast. Add one-half of a thinly cut, ripe avocado to each piece of bread once it has finished cooking. Put one egg on each slice of toast after cooking two eggs according to your preference — scrambled, over-easy, or sunny-side up. Lastly, add salt and pepper to taste and enjoy your toast!

Due to the presence of monounsaturated and omega-3 fatty acids, avocado is a fantastic source of the good fats needed for fertility. These lipids are crucial for optimal ovulation and hormone production. In addition to being a good source of vitamins and minerals including vitamin E, magnesium, and fiber to aid with digestion, avocados also contain

omelet of fertility

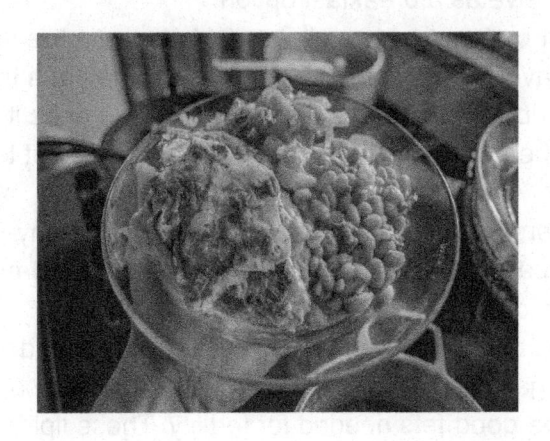

The fertility omelet is a straightforward and delectable recipe that is perfect for breakfast or a light dinner. This meal is a perfect addition to any fertility cookbook for couples because it is loaded with nutrients that are crucial for a healthy reproductive system. Eggs, spinach, onion, mushrooms, and herbs make up the majority of this omelet's ingredients. Protein, folate, and zinc are all essential nutrients for reproductive health and are all abundant in eggs. Vitamin C, an antioxidant that aids in defending the reproductive system against free radical damage, is abundant in spinach.

Furthermore rich in minerals like the B vitamins (B6, B12, and folate), onions and mushrooms are beneficial for reproductive health. Last but not least, herbs like thyme, chives, and parsley offer taste and nutrition. Start by whisking the eggs and herbs in a bowl before making the omelet. Add one tablespoon of oil to a non-stick skillet that is already hot over medium-high heat. Add the mushrooms and onions, and cook until the mushrooms are brown and the onions are tender. After adding, boil the spinach until it wilts. When the eggs are set, pour the egg mixture over the vegetables and simmer. After flipping, cook the omelet for one more minute. With the omelet, offer whole grain bread or fresh fruit.

Oatmeal Parfait

Yogurt parfait is a delectable and healthy alternative for a snack or breakfast for couples trying to get pregnant. It is simple to prepare and rich in healthy nutrients like proteins, vitamins, minerals, probiotics, and good fats. Yogurt is a fantastic source of calcium, which is necessary for strong bones and teeth as well as for hormone regulation. Yogurt's probiotics have been shown to enhance gut health, which is crucial for the wellbeing of both partners.

Start by layering a cup of plain Greek yogurt with any of your preferred fruits, nuts, and seeds to produce a yogurt parfait. Blueberries, raspberries, bananas, walnuts, and chia seeds are a few healthy options. For a little sweetness, you may also add a spoonful of honey or maple syrup. Some granola or oats can be added to the parfait to make it even healthier. Once the parfait is put together, drizzle some honey over it or sprinkle some cinnamon on top.

Yogurt parfait is a delicious and healthy snack that couples trying to get pregnant can enjoy at any time. It is easy to prepare and offers a balanced diet of protein, carbs, and vitamins and minerals to promote a strong reproductive system. It also tastes fantastic! Savor this tasty treat as you move closer to a healthy pregnancy.

Sweet Oatmeal

Savory oatmeal is a satisfying, healthy, and adaptable meal that is ideal for couples trying to get pregnant. This recipe is loaded with complex carbs and fiber, which can help both men and women become more fertile. Zinc, which is essential for conception and fertilization, is abundant in oats. In addition, this dish is a good source of selenium, vitamin B6, iron, and other essential vitamins and minerals that promote reproductive health.

Another excellent method to include a variety of vegetables in your diet is with savory oatmeal. For a flavorful supper, include some cooked spinach, diced tomatoes, mushrooms, onions, and garlic. This dish may be prepared fast and easily, saving busy couples a lot of time.

Boiling the oats in water or vegetable stock for around five minutes is the first step in making savory oatmeal. After the oats have finished cooking, add a tablespoon of olive oil and a few seasonings, including basil, oregano, basil, garlic powder, and salt and pepper to taste. Finally, combine everything after adding your chosen vegetables. Serve after garnishing with some fresh herbs and a drizzle of olive oil.

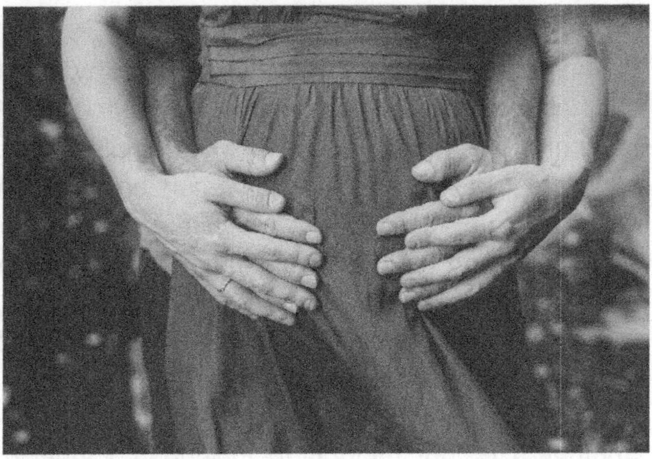

Fertility fruit salad

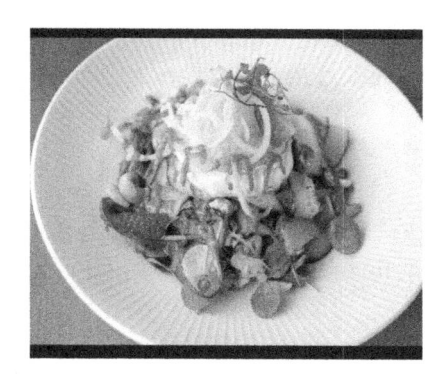

Fertility Fruit Salad is a delicious and healthy way to provide your body with the essential vitamins, minerals, and antioxidants it needs to support healthy fertility. This recipe combines a variety of fruits, nuts, and seeds to create a nutrient-rich salad that can be enjoyed at breakfast, lunch, or dinner.

To make this salad, you will need:

-2 cups fresh seasonal fruit, such as strawberries, blueberries, raspberries, blackberries, diced oranges, diced apples, or diced pears
-1/2 cup chopped walnuts

-1/4 cup dried cranberries
-2 tablespoons flaxseed
-2 tablespoons hemp seeds
-2 tablespoons chia seeds
-1/4 cup freshly squeezed orange juice

Instructions:

1. In a large bowl, combine the fresh fruit, walnuts, cranberries, flaxseed, hemp seeds, and chia seeds.

2. Drizzle the orange juice over the top and mix until all ingredients are evenly coated.

3. Serve the fertility fruit salad immediately, or store it in the refrigerator for up to 3 days.

Enjoy this delicious, nutrient-packed fertility fruit salad as part of a healthy fertility diet!

Breakfast sandwich

For couples trying to increase their chances of getting pregnant, a breakfast sandwich is the perfect option. A breakfast sandwich can give you the energy and nutrition you need to help enhance fertility because it is loaded with protein and nutrients.

Use whole grain breads like rye or whole wheat when assembling a breakfast sandwich that is good for fertility. Complex carbohydrates and fiber found in these breads can assist to control blood sugar levels and lessen insulin resistance. Whole grain breads also contain essential vitamins and minerals like folic acid and iron that are crucial for fertility.

Use wholesome, nutrient-rich products for your breakfast sandwich's filling. Choose lean sources of protein such egg whites, ham, chicken, or turkey. Include some good fats, such as avocado or a thin layer of cream cheese. For an additional dose of nutrients, you can also include some leafy greens like spinach or arugula. Make sure your sandwich has a nutritious spread or condiment. Hummus, nut butters, and avocado spread are all good choices for fertility. Also, you can boost the flavor by using herbs and spices like oregano, basil, and garlic.

The fact that breakfast sandwiches are simple to create and can be tailored to suit your specific nutritional requirements is one of their best features. It's a terrific way to start the day off, whether you decide to prepare it at home or buy a premade sandwich from the shop.

Have
a
magical
Thanksgiving

Pancakes that are sterility-friendly

Couples who are trying to get pregnant frequently struggle to find meals that are both nourishing and delicious. Pancakes may be simply modified to be fertility friendly and are a terrific way to start the day. Couples trying to conceive have a delicious and wholesome food to choose from in this cookbook on fertility.

These pancakes are loaded with nutrients that promote conception. They contain ground flaxseed and chia seeds for extra omega-3 fatty acids as well as whole wheat flour for slow-release energy. Bananas are a good source of potassium and vitamin B6, both of which have been associated with higher female fertility. Protein and calcium, which are crucial for a healthy conception, are also found in milk and yogurt.
These Fertility-Friendly Pancakes are made by:

Ingredients:
- A single cup of whole wheat flour
- 2 tablespoons of flaxseed, ground
- Chia seeds, 2 teaspoons
baking powder, 1 teaspoon

baking soda, 1 teaspoon
Salt, 1/2 teaspoon
- 1 mashed, ripe banana
Yogurt, 1 cup
-1 cup milk
- 2 eggs
honey, 2 tablespoons
- 2 teaspoons melted butter

Instructions:

1. Mix the flour, flaxseed, chia seeds, salt, baking soda, and baking powder in a sizable basin.

2. The mashed banana, yogurt, milk, eggs, honey, and melted butter should all be combined in a different bowl.

3. After adding the liquid components, mix the dry ingredients only until they are barely blended.

4. Butter or coconut oil should be used sparingly to lightly lubricate a non-stick pan before heating it up.

5. Spoon 1/4 cup of the batter into the pan, and heat until the surface bubbles and the edges start to curl.

6. The pancake should cook for an additional minute or two after flipping.

7. Repeat with the remainder of the batter after transferring the cooked pancake to a platter.

The best way to start your day off with a nutrient-rich note is with these fertility-friendly pancakes. Serve as a tasty and filling breakfast with a spoonful of honey or your preferred nut butter.

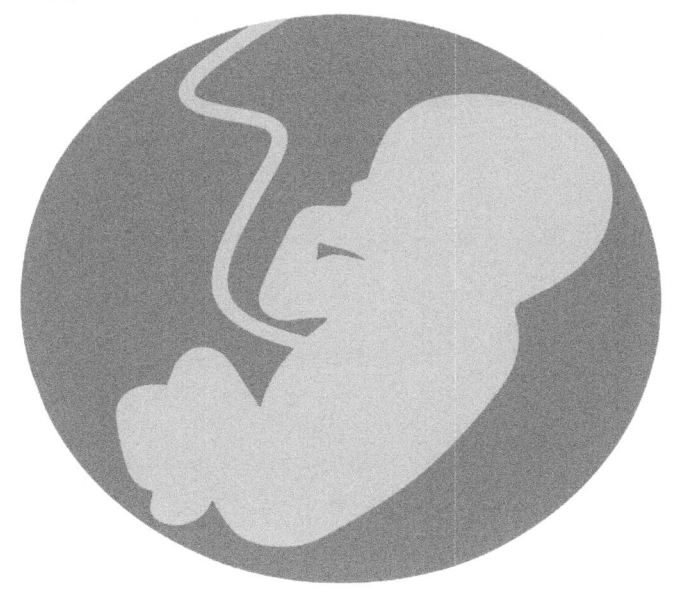

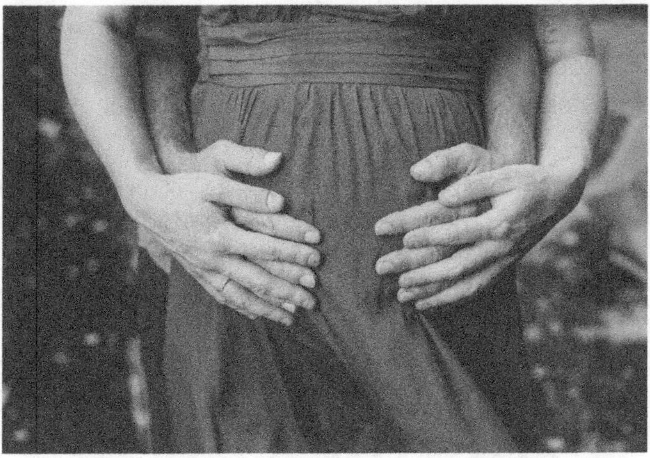

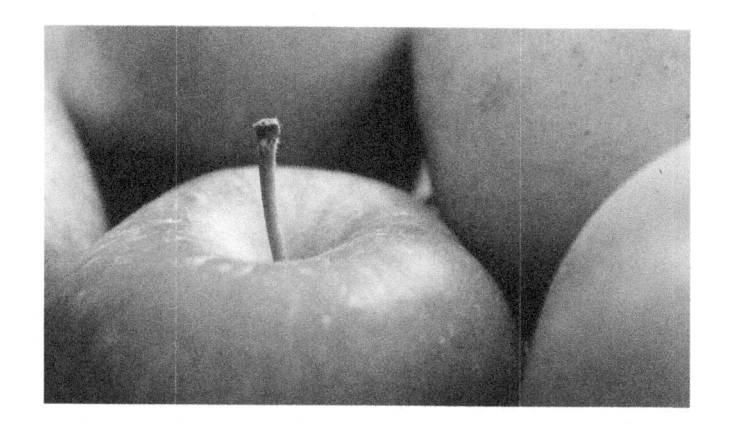

Chapter Four: Lunch

Fertility protein Bowl

The fertility protein bowl is an excellent way for couples to consume the recommended daily intake of protein. These bowls are easy to make, nourishing, and customizable to suit each person's tastes. They are also an excellent way for couples to diversify their diets. A fertility protein bowl often starts with a base of cooked grains, such as quinoa, brown rice, or buckwheat, that are high in protein and other necessary minerals and vitamins. After being seasoned with herbs and spices, these grains can be topped with a variety of vegetables, such as bell peppers, carrots, and mushrooms, as well as foods high in protein, such eggs, beans, nuts, and seeds. Strawberries, blueberries, and raspberries provide a lovely flavor and texture to the bowl. A variety of healthful fats, including tahini, avocado, olive oil, or almonds, can be used as a garnish to a fertility protein bowl. You can also add lemon juice, balsamic vinegar, or various herbs and spices for flavor. Both partners can enjoy a quick and satisfying dinner like a fertility protein bowl. Giving a couple's diet greater variety and nutrition while still providing them with the protein they need to support a healthy reproductive journey might be a great strategy.

fantastic salad

Super salad is a great addition to any cookbook for fertility-conscious couples. It is stuffed with the essential nutrients needed for a strong reproductive system. This salad's combination of ingredients will provide a nourishing and well-balanced lunch for people looking to increase their chances of getting pregnant. The base of the salad is made up of dark leafy greens like spinach, kale, and arugula, which are rich in folic acid, iron, and vitamins A, C, and K. These nutrients are all essential for maintaining hormonal balance and fertility.

You may provide your body the protein, healthy fats, and omega-3 fatty acids it needs for healthy reproduction by including nuts and seeds like walnuts, almonds, and sunflower seeds. These compounds also contain zinc, a mineral that has been linked to improved sperm quality and motility.

Fruit salads including oranges, apples, and berries are wonderful for fertility. They provide vitamin C, which has been linked to improved egg quality and fertility. Berries include a lot of antioxidants as well, which can protect the reproductive system from environmental toxins.

Last but not least, the dish will be topped with a light dressing composed of olive oil, balsamic vinegar, garlic, and herbs to give flavor and additional nutrients like monounsaturated fats and polyphenols. All things considered, a super salad like this one is a great option for couples attempting to conceive more children. Its nutrient-rich components can provide the body with the essential vitamins and minerals required for optimum reproductive health.

Green Wrap

Ingredients:

- Two whole wheat tortillas

2 teaspoons of olive oil

- 12 cups of thinly chopped red onion

- 2 minced cloves of garlic

two cups of kale, chopped

- One cup of cooked quinoa

- One cup of black beans, cooked

- 12 cups chopped bell peppers

- Half a cup of grated carrot

- 1/2 cup crumbled feta cheese

- 1 tablespoon finely chopped fresh parsley

- Two tablespoons of balsamic vinegar

- Salt and black pepper, to taste.

Instructions:

1. In a big skillet, preheat the olive oil over medium heat.
2. The red onion and garlic are added and sautéed for a few minutes until softened.
3. After adding, simmer the kale for 5 minutes, or until wilted.
4. Quinoa, black beans, carrot, bell pepper, feta cheese, and parsley are all added while stirring.
5. Before adding salt and black pepper to taste, sprinkle balsamic vinegar over the mixture.
6. Take from heat and give it a little chance to cool.
7. Spread the veggie mixture over each tortilla after placing them in a row on a work surface.
8. After rolling each tortilla and tucking the ends inside, cut each tortilla in half.
9. Serve warm or at room temperature. Enjoy!

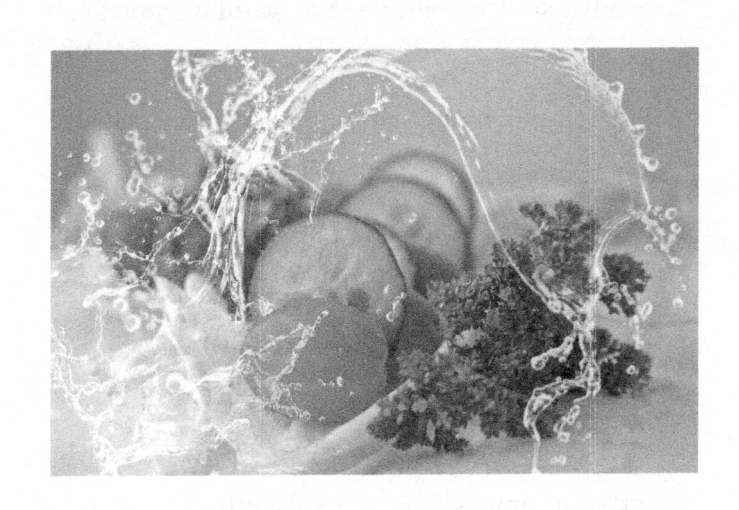

Sandwich with egg salad

For couples trying to conceive, sandwiches with egg salad are a great addition to any cookbook. This recipe is easy to make, packed with protein and healthy fats, and it can be readily modified to suit each person's tastes.

To make an egg salad sandwich, boil a dozen eggs for around 15 minutes. After the eggs have cooled, peel and cube them. In a bowl, combine the eggs, mayonnaise, mustard, salt, and pepper. Use diced celery, red onion, and fresh herbs like dill or parsley for flavor boosts.

Spread the egg salad on the whole wheat bread and top with the pieces of lettuce and tomato. For more crunch, top the sandwich with a couple slices of cucumber or pickle. For a cheesy touch, you can also add more cheese, like Swiss or cheddar. Sandwiches with egg salad are another fantastic breakfast food that is high in protein. Serve the sandwiches with a side of fresh fruit and a glass of milk for a complete dinner.

Bean burger

For couples who are attempting to get pregnant, bean burgers are a great substitute. These filling veggie burgers are an easy-to-make, flavorful dinner that's rich in protein, fiber, and other fertility-boosting ingredients.

In order to make these delicious bean burgers, begin by gathering the following ingredients: 1 can of black beans, 1/2 cup cooked quinoa, 1/2 cup cooked brown rice, 1/2 cup diced onion, 1/4 cup diced red bell pepper, 1/4 cup diced green bell pepper, 1/4 cup diced carrot, 1/4 cup diced celery, 1/4 cup diced mushrooms, and 1/4 cup diced tomatoes.

After that, empty the can of black beans into a big bowl and mash with a fork or a potato masher until a paste forms. After adding the cooked quinoa, rice, veggies, and diced tomatoes, stir everything together thoroughly. Divide the ingredients into six equal amounts and form patties. Finally, put a pan over medium-high heat and add a tablespoon of oil. For golden brown patties, fry them in the pan for 4-5 minutes on each side. Over a bed of lettuce, enjoy the burgers with your favorite dipping sauces.

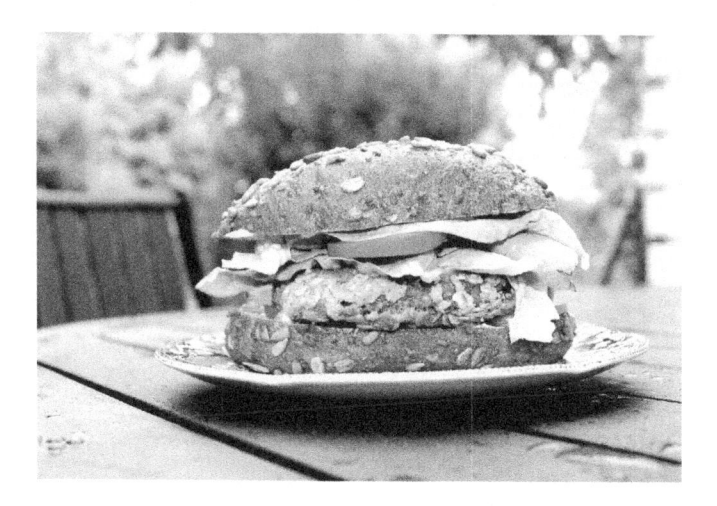

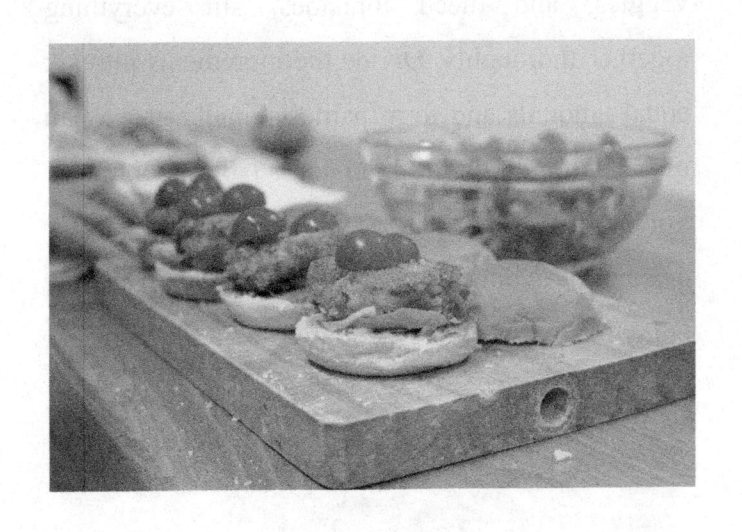

salad with kale and chicken

Chicken and kale salad is a nutritious, mouthwatering food that would be a perfect addition to any cookbook for couples on fertility. Due to its high content of essential vitamins, minerals, essential fatty acids, and fiber, this salad is an excellent choice for those trying to get pregnant.

The salad's base is made of fresh kale, a nutritional powerhouse. Kale has large amounts of calcium, iron, potassium, and the vitamins A, C, and K. Because it is a great source of fiber and antioxidants, it is a fantastic option for women who are trying to get pregnant.

The salad's base is made of fresh kale, a nutritional powerhouse. Kale has large amounts of calcium, iron, potassium, and the vitamins A, C, and K. Because it is a great source of fiber and antioxidants, it is a fantastic option for women who are trying to get pregnant. The salad also contains chicken, which is a great source of protein. Since protein regulates the production of hormones, it is essential for fertility. B vitamins, which are essential for creating energy, are also included in chicken.

To prepare the kale for the salad, cut off the stems and shred the leaf. After thoroughly washing the kale, massage it with some salt and olive oil. As a result, the kale gets softer and more flavorful.

After that, the chicken must be fully cooked. The greens are combined with pieces of chopped chicken. Any extra ingredients you select, like sliced tomatoes, cucumbers, or red onion, should be added last.

After all the ingredients have been combined, dress the salad with a simple vinaigrette made of olive oil, lemon juice, and your preferred herbs. This salad tastes great cold or at room temperature as a side dish or light supper.

Chicken and kale salad is a nutritious dish that's packed with required fatty acids, essential vitamins, and minerals. Due to the fact that it provides them with the nutrition their bodies require, it is a fantastic alternative for couples who are trying to get pregnant.

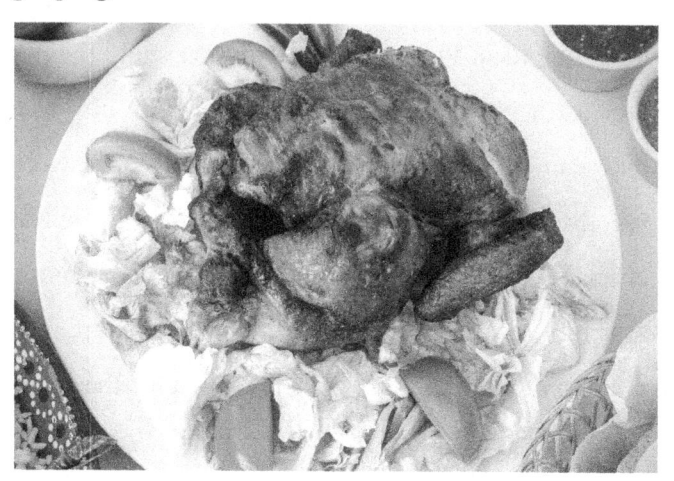

Chapter 5: DINNER

Pumpkin power Salad

For couples searching for a meal that promotes conception, pumpkin power salad is a simple and delicious idea. Pumpkin, kale, quinoa, and almonds are just a few of the healthy nutrients in this salad that can aid with fertility. These nutrients work together to create a complete protein, which is crucial for fertility. Beta-carotene, a vitamin essential for a healthy reproductive system, and vitamins A and C are also abundant in the salad thanks to the addition of pumpkin. Prepare the ingredients first before making the salad. Start by preparing a cup of quinoa per the directions on the package. Place the cooked quinoa aside to cool. Prepare the other ingredients in the meantime. One bunch of washed and roughly chopped kale should be put in a big bowl. One small pumpkin, peeled and chopped, is added to the basin.

Then, add 3 tablespoons of olive oil, 1/4 cup of dried cranberries, and 1/2 cup of chopped pecans to the bowl. Lastly, sprinkle the cooked quinoa on top. Add salt and pepper to taste and toss everything together. Add a dollop of Greek yogurt to the salad to give it a creamy touch. For dinner, this Pumpkin Power Salad is a fantastic choice for a couple trying to conceive. It only takes a few minutes to put together and is packed with nutritious elements that are essential for fertility. Enjoy!

swift salmon

For couples seeking for a dinner that is fertility-friendly, Quick Salmon is a delicious and time-saving choice. This meal can be served as the main course or as a component of a bigger dinner and is quick and simple to prepare. Salmon filet serves as the primary component in Fast Salmon. Omega-3 fatty acids, which are necessary for optimal fertility, are abundant in salmon. The generation of hormones depends on vitamin D, which salmon provides an excellent source of. This quick and simple dish can be made in a matter of minutes, making it the perfect midweek supper.

Set the oven to 400°F before preparing the Quick Salmon. Salt and pepper the salmon filets before placing them on a baking pan lined with parchment paper. Bake for 15 minutes, or until the salmon is thoroughly cooked, in the preheated oven. Prepare a quick sauce to go with the salmon while it bakes. One tablespoon of olive oil is heated to medium heat in a small pan. 1 minced garlic clove, 1 tbsp. honey, 1 tsp. fresh lemon juice, and a dash of sea salt should all be added. Simmer for two minutes while stirring now and then.

Serve the salmon with the sauce after it has finished baking. Serve Quick Salmon with a side of vegetables and a crisp salad for a complete feast. A fantastic, quick dish full of components that are good for fertility is Fast Salmon. Any meal rotation that promotes conception will undoubtedly include this delectable dish on a regular basis.

Reproductive Casserole

A tasty, nutrient-rich dish called fertility casserole is ideal for a romantic night in with your sweetheart or a dinner party. This substantial casserole is a terrific dish for any couple trying to get pregnant because it is full of fertility-friendly components including eggs, spinach, and other vegetables.

In order to prepare a fertility casserole, preheat your oven to 350°F. Then, combine 8 eggs, 1 cup milk, 1 teaspoon dried oregano, and 1 teaspoon garlic powder in a big bowl. Set aside.

1 cup cooked brown rice, 1 cup diced tomatoes, 1 cup chopped spinach, 1 cup diced bell peppers, 1 cup diced onion, 1 cup diced mushrooms, and 1 cup grated cheese should all be combined in a separate bowl. Apply cooking spray to the bottom of an 8-inch casserole dish and top with half of the veggie mixture. Then, add the remaining vegetables on top of the egg mixture. Grated cheese should be added on the casserole's top.

The casserole should be baked for 40 minutes, or until the center is set and the top is golden brown. Before serving, let the dish cool for ten minutes. Enjoy! Including a range of ingredients that are good for conception in your diet is easy with a fertility casserole. The vegetables are brimming with vitamins, minerals, and antioxidants that are crucial for a healthy reproductive system, while the eggs offer protein and key vitamins. The brown rice offers fiber and complex carbohydrates, while the cheese offers heart-healthy fats.

For a well-rounded supper, eat this fertility casserole with a side salad or vegetable soup. Don't forget dessert, either! After a meal that promotes fertility, a piece of dark chocolate or a cup of frozen yogurt may be the ideal dessert.

Filling Chicken

A traditional dish like stuffed chicken can be a tasty, filling, and simple supper for couples who are trying to conceive. It might be a fantastic method to add more protein, good fats, and necessary vitamins and minerals to your diet. You must first choose the proper variety of chicken before you can proceed. Because they are lean and loaded with protein, chicken breasts are a great option. You may also use chicken thighs, which have more fat but are still healthy.

Once you've decided on your chicken, you can start stuffing it. The chicken should first be butterflied, which entails cutting it horizontally to make a pocket for the stuffing. The pocket can then be filled with your preferred ingredients. Cooked rice, prepared veggies, and herbs & spices are a few examples. For more flavor and nutrition, you can also add cheese, almonds, or other nutritious items.

Depending on the size of the chicken, after stuffing it, you can secure it with toothpicks, wrap it in parchment paper, and bake it for 25 to 30 minutes. Before eating, make sure the chicken is fully cooked.

Given that it is so full of nutrients necessary for a healthy reproductive system, stuffed chicken is a fantastic dinner for couples who are concerned about their ability to conceive. The energy and nourishment required for fertility can be helped by eating a variety of lean proteins, healthy fats, and complex carbohydrates. Also, incorporating herbs and spices into your food might help you consume more antioxidants, which can protect cells from deterioration and enhance general health.

Seafood Stew

Oyster stew is a robust and delicious dish that can give couples trying to conceive a filling and delectable evening. By including nutrient-rich components like fish, veggies, and herbs, it is a fantastic approach to boost fertility.

Start by sautéing some veggies, such as celery, onions, and garlic, in a big pot before making oyster stew for dinner. Add a few tablespoons of butter and let it melt after the vegetables have softened. Add two pints of shucked oysters and some white wine after that. Add some fresh herbs like parsley and thyme after the first five minutes of simmering. Add salt and pepper to taste after simmering for a further 15 minutes.

Pour the stew into individual bowls once it has finished cooking and sprinkle with freshly grated parmesan cheese. Rice or crusty bread should be served alongside it. Due to its abundance of fertility-boosting minerals, oyster stew is a fantastic choice for couples attempting to conceive. Zinc, which is necessary for good sperm production and ovulation, is found in abundance in oysters. Moreover, they contain a lot of omega-3 fatty acids, which can assist to balance hormones. The stew's veggies and herbs also include vitamins and minerals that may improve fertility.

Overall, a healthy and mouth watering supper option for couples trying to get pregnant is oyster stew. It is simple to prepare and packed with nutrients that can increase fertility. Enjoy!

Chapter 6: Desserts and Drinks

Desserts

Pumpkin pie

One of the most popular fall desserts is pumpkin pie. It is a nutrient-dense dessert that would make a wonderful addition to any cookbook for couples looking to get pregnant. Pumpkin puree is the major component in pumpkin pie. The nutrients in this puree are abundant and crucial for fertility. It is an excellent source of vitamins A and C, which are crucial for reproductive health, as well as beta-carotene, which aids in the body's ability to turn food into energy. Pumpkin also has a lot of fiber, which can balance hormones and help control blood sugar levels.

Moreover, pumpkin pie is quite adaptable. It can be used as a savory dish, dessert, or even for breakfast. Making a breakfast out of pumpkin pie can help couples who want to increase their fertility. Eggs, pumpkin puree, and other nutritious components like nuts, seeds, and spices can be combined to make the filling. The filling can be sweetened by mixing brown sugar, cinnamon, and nutmeg if couples want to make a dessert. In terms of the crust, you can use a graham cracker crust or a classic pastry crust to make pumpkin pie. All selections are delectable and packed with nutritious components. Make the crust with whole wheat flour and use less sugar for a healthy alternative. Any fertility cookbook for couples should include pumpkin pie. It is not only a dessert that is rich in nutrients, but it is also adaptable, offering both savory and sweet possibilities. Many of the components in pumpkin pie are good for fertility, and eating it can be a fantastic way to acquire more of the vitamins and minerals your body needs.

Nut Cake

A simple yet delectable recipe called "Nut Cake" is sure to entice the taste buds of infertile couples. This traditional cake has everything you need to encourage fertility and aid in conception.

Nuts, fruits, and spices are combined to create this cake. Nuts are exceptionally rich in zinc, which is good for fertility in both men and women. Zinc increases the likelihood of ovulation in women and helps males produce more sperm. Figs and dates are a great addition to this cake because they both contain zinc.

Nut Cake also includes a range of spices, including cinnamon, nutmeg, and cardamom, in addition to these components. These spices are well recognized for promoting fertility because they promote circulation and blood sugar regulation.

To create this cake, combine all the ingredients in a basin, and then pour the mixture into a greased cake pan. The cake is then baked for 45 minutes at 375 degrees Fahrenheit. Let the cake cool once baking is complete before cutting and serving.

Any cookbook for couples on fertility should include nuts cake. It is a delectable treat that will undoubtedly improve fertility and raise the likelihood of conception. It will be a hit with any couple trying to conceive thanks to its delectable component mix.

Brownies

Brownies are a tasty and well-liked dish that can be included in a cookbook for couples on fertility. Due to the fact that they can be prepared jointly in the kitchen and savored as a special treat, brownies are a terrific method to involve both couples in the fertility journey. Brownies are an excellent option for a fertility cookbook because they frequently contain lots of taste and minerals. A range of nutrient-rich ingredients, including whole wheat flour, oats, almonds, and dark chocolate, are used in many brownie recipes. A diet rich in nutrients and balanced with these elements can encourage healthy fertility. Moreover, brownies contain a lot of dark chocolate, which is a fantastic source of antioxidants that may help prevent oxidative stress, a factor that may affect fertility.

Couples on the fertility path may find a lot of solace and delight in brownies. Celebrating the minor wins can keep partners motivated, and sharing a tasty treat can be a good way to take a break from the process' tension.

It's crucial to remember to limit amounts if you want to include brownies in your fertility cookbook. Brownies can be a high-calorie treat, so it's crucial to keep your intake in check. However, there are other recipes that swap out some of the more calorie-dense ingredients, like butter and sugar, with healthy alternatives, including Greek yogurt and dates, for those seeking a healthier version of brownies.

Overall, brownies can be a wonderful addition to a cookbook for couples looking to conceive. They are a delightful treat that can give both lovers a much-needed moment of happiness and solace as well as a nutrient-dense, fertility-supporting meal.

Fruit Cheesecake

Berry cheesecake is a rich, delectable dessert that would make a wonderful addition to any fertility recipe book for couples. It is a lovely way to recognize the important event of becoming parents as well as the impending addition to the family.
A sweet, creamy cheesecake baked with a selection of fresh berries makes up this delicious treat. A mouthwatering treat is created when the sweetness of the berries perfectly balances the cheesecake's creaminess. You will need cream cheese, sugar, eggs, and a variety of fresh berries to make the cheesecake. Set the oven to 350 degrees to begin. Then, combine the cream cheese, sugar, and eggs in

a bowl and stir until the mixture is creamy and smooth.

The cream cheese mixture should be distributed in a buttered 9-inch springform pan. Bake the dish in the oven for 30 minutes, or until the middle is firm. Let the cheesecake cool completely after baking it before sprinkling it with fresh berries. The berries should be washed, chopped into little pieces, and then arranged on top of the cheesecake after it has cooled. Put the pan in the fridge and give the cheesecake at least two hours to chill.

Remove the cheesecake from the pan when it's time to serve, then top it with more fresh berries. Take advantage of this delectable berry cheesecake as a special treat to celebrate starting a family. It will surely please even the pickiest of palates thanks to its sweet, creamy flavor and profusion of fresh berries. Enjoy!

dessert made with sweet potatoes

For couples hoping to boost their fertility, sweet potato cheesecake is the ideal treat. It not only gives a tasty pleasure, but it also has a lot of fertility-enhancing advantages. Beta-carotene, which is abundant in sweet potatoes and helps to balance reproductive hormones, raises a couple's chances of getting pregnant. Also, sweet potatoes include vital nutrients including folate, which is crucial for a baby's development.

It's crucial to utilize top-notch ingredients while cooking a sweet potato cheesecake. Beginning with a graham cracker and butter base will aid in holding the cake together. After that, pick the best sweet potatoes you can. Before including the potatoes in the batter, take sure to peel and mash them. You

74

could also add some cream cheese or ricotta cheese to the mixture for a deeper flavor.

When the batter is prepared, place it into a springform pan that has been preheated and bake it until the center is firm. Let the cheesecake cool entirely before serving once it is finished baking. Add some whipped cream or your preferred fruit on top to complete it.

The perfect dessert for couples trying to increase their fertility is sweet potato cheesecake. In addition to being tasty and simple to prepare, it also offers vital nutrients to promote a healthy pregnancy. Savor this delectable delicacy and let it strengthen your bond as a family as you work toward your objectives.

Reproductive cookies

Cookies for fertility are a tasty and healthy snack that can support infertile couples. They are especially useful for ladies who want to become more fertile. Ingredients in fertility cookies have the potential to encourage the synthesis of hormones that are crucial for conceiving a child. Many ingredients can be used to make these cookies. Oats, barley, and quinoa are some whole grains that are excellent providers of fiber, support a healthy digestive system, and maintain stable blood sugar levels. As they include omega-3 fatty acids and other necessary minerals and vitamins, nuts, seeds, and nut butters are also a fantastic addition to fertility cookies. Fruits like apricots, apples, and bananas can be added to diets to help supply essential vitamins and minerals for fertility.

Honey is the ideal ingredient to use when sweetening the cookies. A natural sweetener recognized for its antibacterial and antimicrobial properties, honey can help increase fertility. The addition of herbs like nettle and red raspberry leaves can also aid to support a healthy reproductive system.

Fertility cookies are a delicious morning or afternoon snack that may be eaten at any time of the day. These cookies can also be preserved for up to five days in the refrigerator in an airtight container.

DRINKS

Ovulation smoothie with blueberries

A delicious, wholesome, and simple-to-make smoothie called a blueberry ovulation smoothie can help couples improve their chances of getting pregnant. This smoothie is loaded with nutrients that promote conception and good ovulation. It has blueberries, which are believed to help balance hormones and increase fertility because they are rich in antioxidants and fiber. Greek yogurt, which is a rich source of calcium and protein necessary for healthy ovulation and fertility, is also included in the smoothie. It also has flaxseed, which is high in omega-3 fatty acids and has the ability to balance hormones. Last but not least, it contains honey, a natural sweetener rich in vitamins and minerals that can also increase fertility.

Any fertility cookbook for couples would benefit greatly from the addition of this blueberry ovulation smoothie. It's not only tasty and healthy, but it's also simple to make. A blender, a few ingredients, and a few minutes of your time are all you need. This smoothie can also be prepared in advance and kept in the refrigerator so you can enjoy it whenever you want a quick, wholesome snack or beverage.

This ovulation smoothie with blueberries is simple to make. Blueberries, Greek yogurt, flaxseed, and honey must all be put in a blender and blend until smooth. You can also add a little cinnamon or nutmeg if you want to boost the flavor. After the smoothie has been blended, pour some into a glass and sip it.

Overall, a fertility menu for couples would benefit greatly from including this blueberry ovulation smoothie. In addition to being filling and simple to prepare, it can also help couples improve their chances of getting pregnant. So why not give it a shot and see if it aids in your fertility objectives?

shake with protein and peanut butter

A fantastic meal to aid couples attempting to conceive is the peanut butter protein smoothie from the couples' fertility cookbook. This recipe makes a delightful smoothie that can increase fertility by fusing the protein-rich benefits of peanut butter with the health advantages of fruits and vegetables. Couples can easily consume more of the vitamins and minerals necessary for reproductive health thanks to the smoothie's natural sweetness.

Beginning with 1 cup of almond milk, combine the Peanut Butter Protein Smoothie for Fertility Cookbook for Couples. Add 1 banana, 1/4 cup peanut butter, 1/2 cup each of frozen blueberries and strawberries following that. The components should be smooth after being blended. To sweeten the smoothie, you can choose to add a teaspoon of honey or a tablespoon of maple syrup.

Pour the smoothie into two glasses when it has been mixed. The smoothie is prepared for consumption. This dish offers a fantastic source of the vitamins, minerals, and protein needed for fertility. Also, it offers a delightful and wholesome way to start the day. Add a scoop of protein powder to the smoothie to increase its nutritional content if you want to acquire more of the vitamins and minerals necessary for fertility. A handful of spinach or kale will also offer extra vitamins, minerals, and antioxidants to the smoothie that can boost reproductive health.

A fantastic meal for couples attempting to get pregnant is the peanut butter protein smoothie from the couples' fertility cookbook. It offers a tasty approach to receive the vitamins and minerals necessary for fertility as well as a fantastic protein source. Use this smoothie as a snack or a breakfast meal substitute.

CONCLUSION

Finally, the fertility cookbook for couples is a priceless tool for those trying to conceive. The recipes, information, and techniques it offers can help couples increase their chances of getting pregnant. Also, it provides a selection of healthy meals that are intended to keep both couples strong and healthy throughout the conception process. Couples can collaborate to produce a wholesome, balanced diet that will support their fertility objectives by adhering to these recommendations and recipes. Couples who have the necessary information, commitment, and determination can fulfill their ambition of becoming parents.